Quality measures associated with the Minimum Data Set (MDS) in the Resident Assessment Instrument (RAI)

How nursing homes can avoid common calculation errors

Anna May Xu

Table of contents

Chapter 1: Introduction

All skilled nursing facilities (SNFs) that participate in Medicare or Medicaid have to periodically collect and submit statistics about how well they're running their organizations to the Centers for Medicare & Medicaid Services (CMS). These measurements are called **quality measures**, or **QMs**. You can have quality measures for pretty much anything that goes on in the nursing home: staffing levels, number of residents who have particular diseases, mortality rates, etc.

In the olden days, people had to manually extract data from the paper clinical record. But now, data can be automatically extracted from the electronic medical record. Various aspects of clinical care are coded into a standardized set of data elements called the **minimum data set**, or **MDS**. All the data from all the nursing homes in the United States go into national databases. Right now, the MDS data go into the **Quality Improvement and Evaluation System (QIES)** and the **Assessment Submission and Processing (ASAP)** databases, but CMS is working on consolidating those into one big database.

Public reporting of quality measures

Some quality measures are publicly reported to help consumers select a nursing home. These QMs are summarized into a 1-to-5-star rating, with 5 stars being excellent and one star being bad.

Care Compare replaces Nursing Home Compare

Before 2020, Nursing Home Compare was the website where people accessed the 5-star ratings, but the CMS changed it to **Care Compare**. They've consolidated data on physicians, hospitals, nursing homes, home health services, hospices, and dialysis centers. You can also download the data.

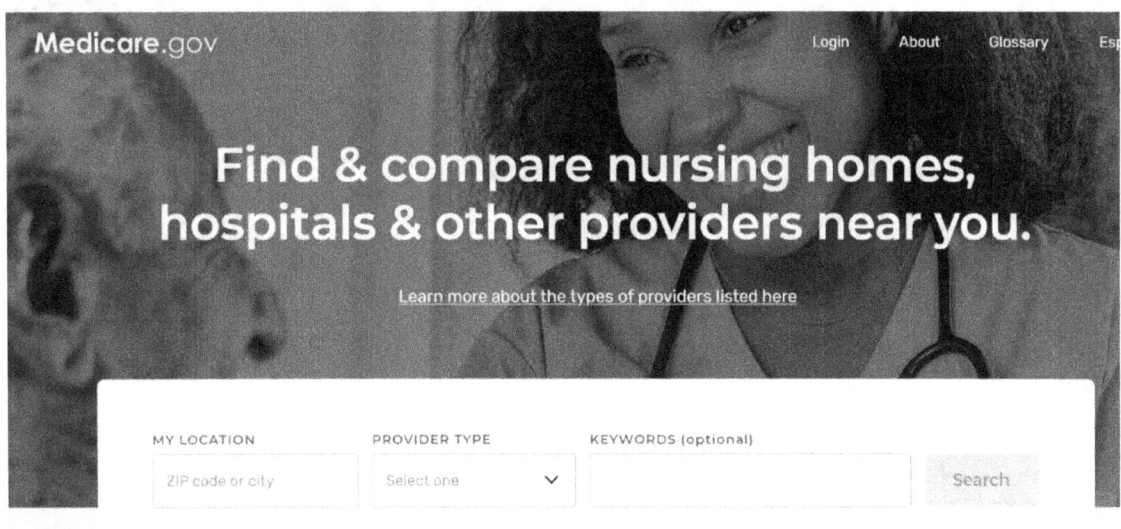

https://www.medicare.gov/care-compare/

Quality Improvement and Evaluation System (QIES)

The **Quality Improvement and Evaluation System**, or **QIES**, is the portal for submitting minimum data set information to the Centers for Medicare and Medicaid Services. Here are the general steps for MDS data submission:

1. Go to the **QIES Technical Support Office** (**QTSO**) website. Click on the CMSNet – Submission Access button.

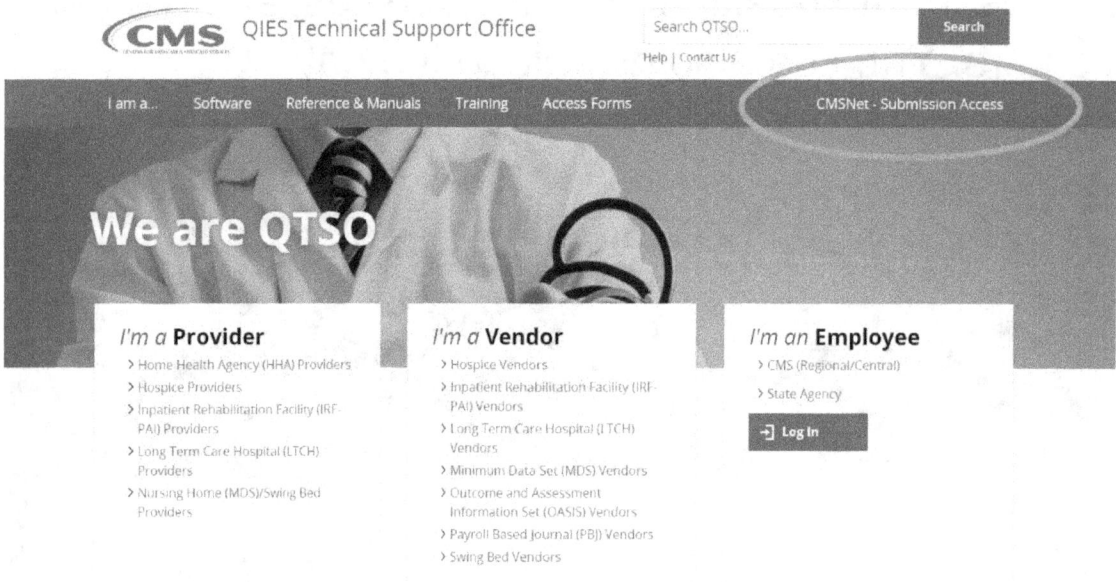

https://qtso.cms.gov/

2. Click on the state that your nursing home is in. I'm from Texas, so I would click TX. You can use the dropdown menu or click on the map.

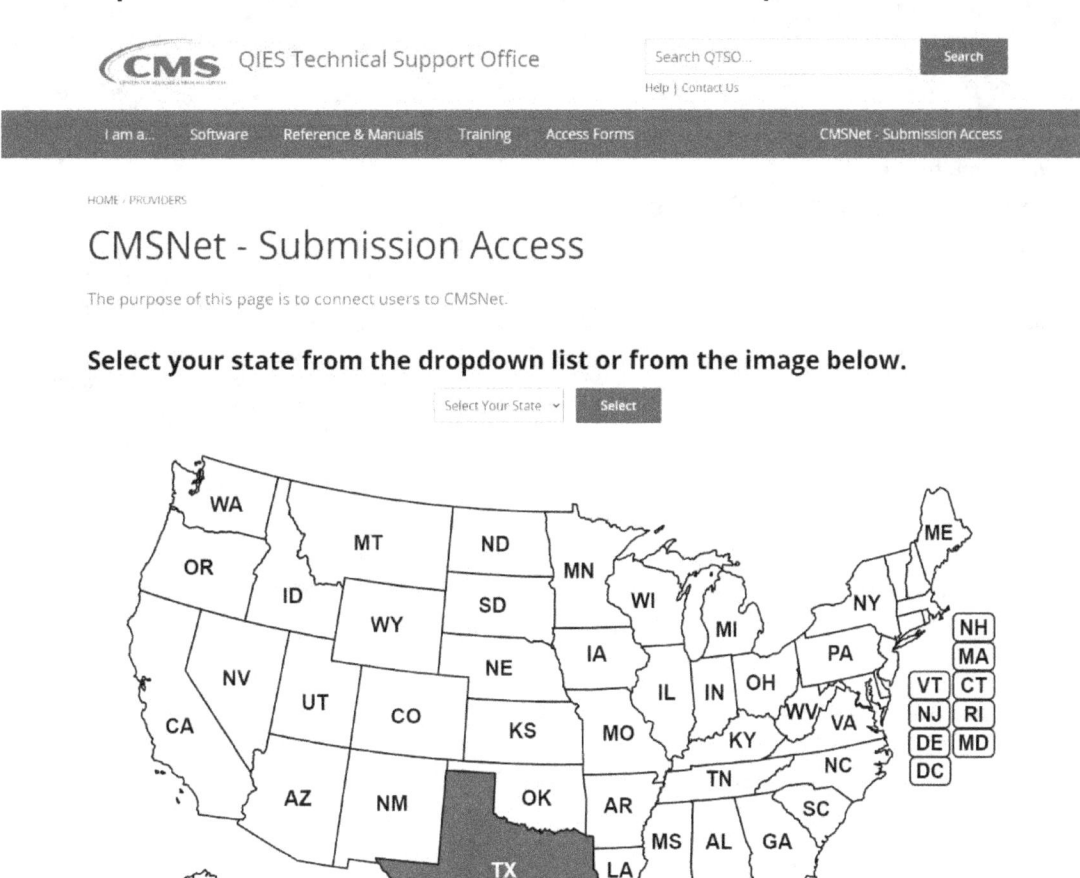

3. Log on to the CMS MDS website. Now you can start submitting MDS data!

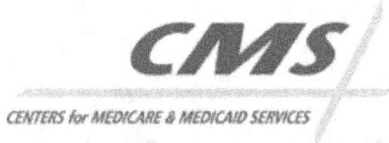

CENTERS for MEDICARE & MEDICAID SERVICES

Welcome to the
CMS Secure Access Service

username [   ]

password [   ]

[Sign In]

NOTE: If this is your first time connecting, you will need to have admin rights to enable the necessary components for remote access to the QIES application. If you do not have admin rights, please contact your local support. If you are having trouble with the password on this page, please contact the CMSNet Helpdesk at (888) 238-2122 https://qtso.cms.gov/cmsnet.html

internet Quality Improvement and Evaluation System (iQIES)

In 2020, CMS debuted a system called the **internet Quality Improvement and Evaluation System (iQIES)** for collecting healthcare data from nursing homes. iQIES will eventually replace and consolidate the QIES, CASPER and ASPEN systems. They're still conducting pilot studies on iQIES, so for now, we still have the big three.

The CASPER system

Nursing homes use the **Certification and Survey Provider Enhanced Reports** (**CASPER**) system to access their quality measure reports.

How to access CASPER

Once you've logged into the CMS MDS system, click on the CASPER Reporting link. This will take you to CASPER.

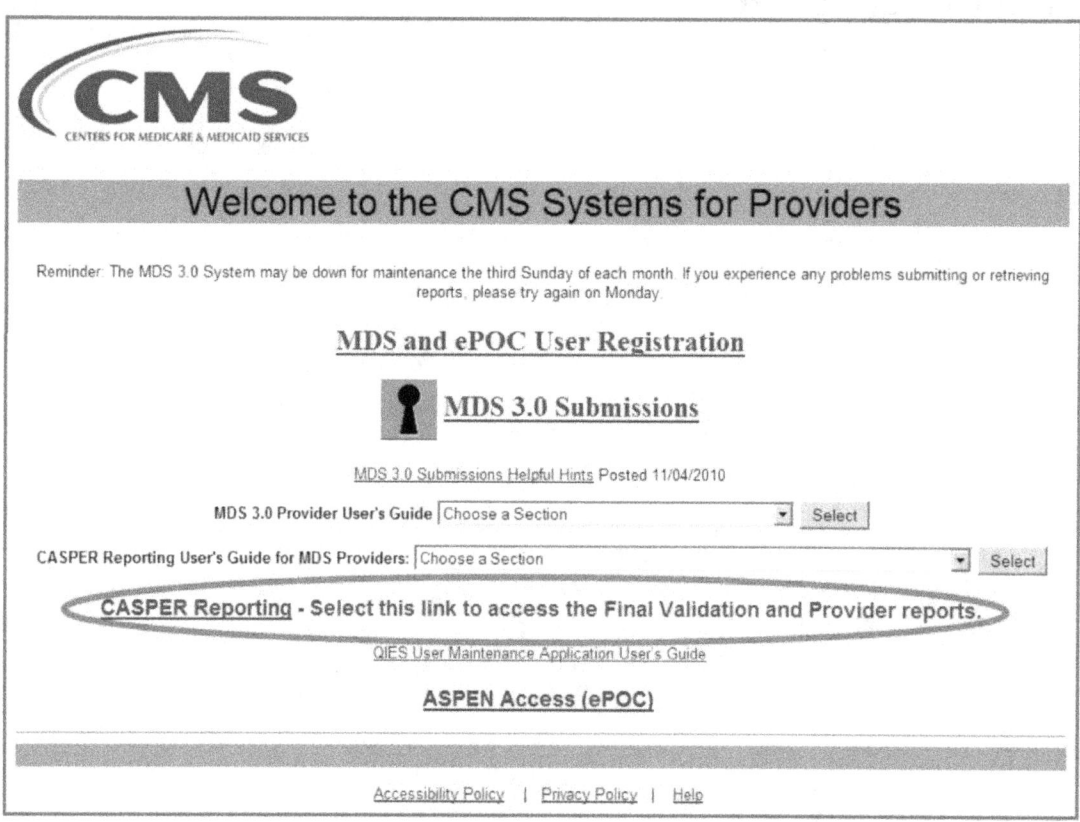

Once you're in CASPER, you can click Reports to see the reports.

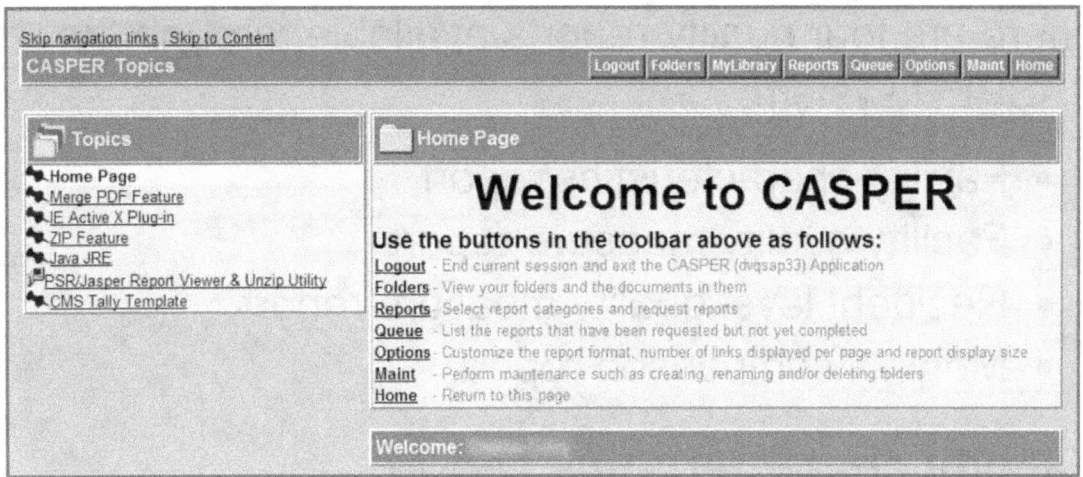

Chapter 2: Quality measure reports

There are four quality reports available through the CASPER system:

- Facility characteristics report
- Facility quality measure report
- Resident level quality measure report
- Monthly comparison report

Facility characteristics report

The facility characteristics report shows demographic information about the nursing home's residents. On CASPER, you can specify various criteria like start date, end date, and comparison group.

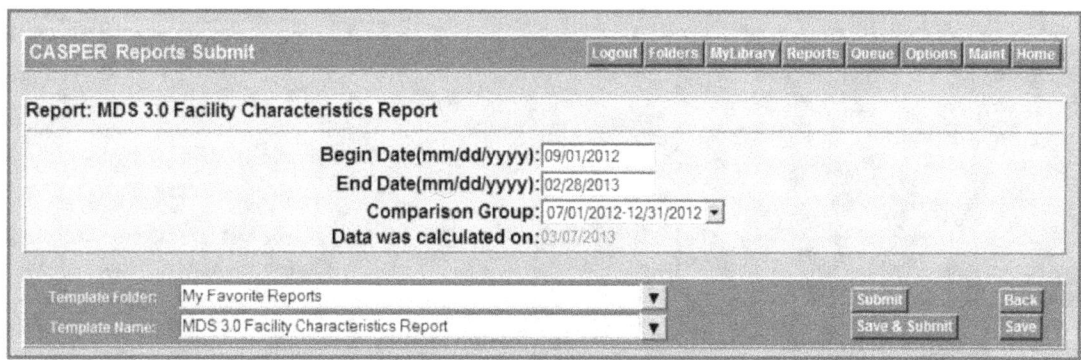

When state comes, they use this report to find resident groups that they want to concentrate on. They might take a closer look at residents who have these kinds of characteristics:

- very old
- male
- have a psychiatric illness, intellectual disability, or developmental disability
- are in hospice
- are newly admitted

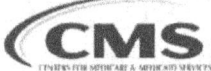

Facility ID: ████████
CCN: ████████
Facility Name: ████████████████
City/State: ████████████

Report Period: 01/01/2020 - 06/30/2020
Comparison Group: 01/01/2020 - 06/30/2020
Report Run Date: 06/01/2020
Data Calculation Date: 10/02/2020
Report Version Number: 1.01

	Facility			Comparison Group	
	Num	Denom	Observed Percent	State Average	National Average
Gender					
Male	898	1,796	50.0%	50.0%	71.5%
Female	898	1,796	50.0%	50.0%	28.5%
Age					
<25 years old	5	1,796	0.3%	0.3%	2.2%
25-54 years old	12	1,796	0.7%	0.7%	0.2%
55-64 years old	57	1,796	3.2%	3.2%	13.5%
65-74 years old	1,558	1,796	86.7%	86.7%	56.8%
75-84 years old	147	1,796	8.2%	8.2%	27.0%
85+ years old	17	1,796	0.9%	0.9%	0.2%
Diagnostic Characteristics					
Psychiatric diagnosis	6	1,785	0.3%	0.3%	3.0%
Intellectual or Developmental Disability	371	371	100.0%	100.0%	75.0%
Hospice	3	1,788	0.2%	0.2%	0.0%
Prognosis					
Life expectancy of less than 6 months	3	1,788	0.2%	0.2%	0.0%
Discharge Plan					
Not already occurring	0	1,796	0.0%	0.0%	25.0%
Already occurring	1,796	1,796	100.0%	100.0%	75.0%
Referral					
Not needed	0	1,796	0.0%	0.0%	25.0%
Is or may be needed but not yet made	0	1,796	0.0%	0.0%	0.0%
Has been made	1,796	1,796	100.0%	100.0%	75.0%
Type of Entry					
Admission	1,795	1,796	99.9%	99.9%	100.0%
Reentry	1	1,796	0.1%	0.1%	0.0%
Entered Facility From					
Community	1,796	1,796	100.0%	100.0%	89.7%
Another nursing home	0	1,796	0.0%	0.0%	1.5%
Acute Hospital	0	1,796	0.0%	0.0%	0.0%
Psychiatric Hospital	0	1,796	0.0%	0.0%	0.0%
Inpatient Rehabilitation Facility	0	1,796	0.0%	0.0%	0.0%
ID/DD facility	0	1,796	0.0%	0.0%	0.0%
Hospice	0	1,796	0.0%	0.0%	0.0%
Long Term Care Hospital	0	1,796	0.0%	0.0%	8.8%
Other	0	1,796	0.0%	0.0%	0.0%

16

The facility characteristics report has two main columns: (1) the facility and (2) the comparison group. Both of them use data for a specified period of time.

The **facility group** has a **numerator**, **denominator**, and **observed percent**. The facility characteristic metrics uses all residents, both short-stay and long-stay residents.

> The numerator is the number of residents with the identified characteristic.

> The denominator is the number of residents in the facility.

> The observed percent is a simple average for each resident characteristic.

The **comparison group** has the **state average** and the **national average**.

> The state average uses data from all facilities in the state.

> The national average uses data from all facilities in the nation.

The facility characteristics report uses the following resident characteristics:

- Gender
    - o Male
    - o Female
- Age
    - o <25 years old
    - o 25-54 years old
    - o 55-64 years old
    - o 65-74 years old
    - o 75-84 years old
    - o 85+ years old
- Diagnostic characteristics
    - o Psychiatric diagnosis
    - o Intellectual or developmental disability
    - o Hospice
- Prognosis
    - o Life expectancy of less than 6 months
- Discharge plan
    - o Not already occurring
    - o Already occurring
- Referral
    - o Not needed
    - o Is or may be needed but not yet made
    - o Has been made

- Type of entry
    - Admission
    - Reentry
- Entered facility from
    - Community
    - Another nursing home
    - Acute hospital
    - Psychiatric hospital
    - Inpatient rehabilitation facility
    - ID/DD facility
    - Hospice
    - Long term care hospital
    - Other

Facility quality measure report

The facility quality measure report shows each quality measure, the numerator and denominator used to compute those quality measures, and how your facility compares to others in the state and in the nation.

The quality metrics are calculated only weekly since the previous week's data collection. That means that if the facility ran the quality metric reports twice in one week, the score would be the same because the data wouldn't have changed.

The state and national comparison group data are only calculated monthly on the first day of the month. Additionally, the data is delayed by 2 months to give people time as a buffer for assessments that are late and need corrections.

The facility quality measure report has 10 columns:

1. the quality measures
2. the quality measures' identification number
3. data

The other seven columns are mathematical calculations:

4. numerator
5. denominator
6. facility observed percent
7. facility adjusted percent
8. comparison group state average
9. comparison group national average
10.   comparison group national percentile

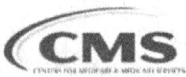
Facility ID:
CCN:
Facility Name:
City/State:

Report Period: 04/01/2021 - 09/30/2021
Comparison Group: 04/01/2021 - 09/30/2021
Report Run Date: 10/01/2021
Data Calculation Date: 10/04/2021
Report Version Number: 3.03

Note: Dashes represent a value that could not be computed
Note: S = short stay, L = long stay
Note: C = complete; data available for all days selected, I = incomplete; data not available for all days selected
Note: * is an indicator used to identify that the measure is flagged
Note: For the Improvement in Function (S) Measure, a single * indicates a Percentile of 25 or less (higher Percentile values are better)

Measure Description	CMS ID	Data	Num	Denom	Facility Observed Percent	Facility Adjusted Percent	Comparison Group State Average	Comparison Group National Average	Comparison Group National Percentile
Hi-risk/Unstageable Pres Ulcer (L)	N015.03	C	0	16	0.0%	0.0%	0.0%	0.0%	0
Phys restraints (L)	N027.02	C	0	53	0.0%	0.0%	0.0%	0.0%	0
Falls (L)	N032.02	C	0	53	0.0%	0.0%	0.0%	0.0%	0
Falls w/Maj Injury (L)	N013.02	C	0	53	0.0%	0.0%	0.0%	0.0%	0
Antipsych Med (S)	N011.02	C	0	0	-	-	-	-	-
Antipsych Med (L)	N031.03	C	53	53	100.0%	100.0%	100.0%	100.0%	100 *
Antianxiety/Hypnotic Prev (L)	N033.02	C	53	53	100.0%	100.0%	100.0%	100.0%	100 *
Antianxiety/Hypnotic % (L)	N036.02	C	53	53	100.0%	100.0%	100.0%	100.0%	100 *
Behav Sx affect Others (L)	N034.02	C	0	53	0.0%	0.0%	0.0%	0.0%	0
Depress Sx (L)	N030.02	C	53	53	100.0%	100.0%	100.0%	100.0%	100 *
UTI (L)	N024.02	C	0	16	0.0%	0.0%	0.0%	0.0%	0
Cath Insert/Left Bladder (L)	N026.03	C	0	16	0.0%	-	-	-	-
Lo-Risk Lose B/B Con (L)	N025.02	C	0	16	0.0%	0.0%	0.0%	0.0%	0
Excess Wt Loss (L)	N029.02	C	16	16	100.0%	100.0%	100.0%	100.0%	100 *
Incr ADL Help (L)	N028.02	C	0	0	-	-	-	-	-
Move Indep Worsens (L)	N035.03	C	0	0	-	-	-	-	-
Improvement in Function (S)	N037.03	C	0	0	-	-	-	-	-

Measure Description	CMS ID	Numerator	Denominator	Facility Observed Percent	Facility Adjusted Percent	National Average
Pressure Ulcer/Injury[1]	S038.02	94	4,748	2.0%	1.2%	0.2%

[1] The Changes in Skin Integrity Post-Acute Care: Pressure Ulcer/Injury (S038.02) measure is calculated using the SNF QRP measure specifications v3.0 addendum and is based on 12 months of data (10/01/2020 - 09/30/2021).

22

Data

In the data column, the letters C and I indicate whether a measure was active during the selected report period.

- **C (complete)**: data available during entire selected period
- **I (incomplete)**: data was not available during the entire selected period

Numerator

The numerator column is the top number of a fraction. It represents the number of residents who had the quality measure condition in the reporting period.

Denominator

The denominator column is the bottom number of a fraction. It represents the number of residents whose assessments were evaluated for presence of the quality measure condition. Some quality measures use a subgroup of total assessed residents.

Facility observed percent

The facility observed percent is the percentage of residents with a quality measure condition. This score is for quality measures that are not risk adjusted.

$$\text{Facility observed percent} = \frac{\text{Numerator}}{\text{denominator}} \times 100$$

Facility adjusted percent

The facility adjusted percent is the facility observed percent that has a risk adjustment applied to it.

Comparison group state average

The comparison group state average is the average of the quality measure percentages for all nursing homes in the state.

Comparison group national average

The comparison group national average is the average of the quality measure percentages for all nursing homes in the nation.

Comparison group national percentile

The comparison group national percentile is the nursing home's rank relative to all other nursing homes in the nation. The percentile rank represents the percentage of facilities that score better than your facility. For example, a nursing home with a 40th percentile rank has a better score than 60% of the nursing homes in the nation. Any metric with a 75th percentile rank or higher automatically gets that metric put under review.

Resident level quality measure report

The resident level quality report shows all residents who were included in the quality measure calculations. It includes both active and discharged residents. This number is the same as the numerator of the calculations in the facility quality measure report.

CMS
CENTERS FOR MEDICARE & MEDICAID SERVICES

CASPER Report
MDS 3.0 Resident Level Quality Measure Report
Page 21 of 498

Facility ID:
Facility Name:
CCN:
City/State:

Report Period: 04/01/2021 - 09/30/2021
Report Run Date: 10/07/2021
Data Calculation Date: 10/04/2021
Report Version Number: 3.03

Note: **S** = short stay, **L** = long stay, **X** = triggered, **b** = not triggered or excluded.
C = complete; data available for all days selected, **I** = incomplete; data not available for all days selected

Resident Name	Resident ID	A0310A/B/F	Hi-risk/Unstageable Pres Ulcer (L)	Phys restraints (L)	Falls (L)	Falls w/Maj Injury (L)	Antipsych Med (S)	Antipsych Med (L)	Antianxiety/Hypnotic Prev (L)	Antianxiety/Hypnotic (L)	Behav Sx Affect Others (L)	Depress Sx (L)	UTI (L)	Cath Insert/Left Bladder (L)	Lo-Risk Lose B/B Con (L)	Excess Wt Loss (L)	Incr ADL Help (L)	Move Indep Worsens (L)	Improvement in Function (S)	Quality Measure Count
Data			C	C	C	C	C	C	C	C	C	C	C	C	C	C	C	C	C	0
Active Residents																				
	48207520	04/99/99	b	b	b	b	b	b	b	b	b	b	b	b	b	b	b	b	b	0
	48207523	05/99/99	b	b	b	b	b	b	b	b	b	b	b	b	b	b	b	b	b	0
	48207526	02/99/99	b	b	b	b	b	b	b	b	b	b	b	b	b	b	b	b	b	0
	48207529	06/99/99	b	b	b	b	b	X	X	X	b	X	b	b	b	X	b	b	b	5
	48207532	99/01/99	b	b	b	b	b	X	X	X	b	X	b	b	b	b	b	b	b	4
	48207535	01/99/99	b	b	b	b	b	X	X	X	b	X	b	b	b	b	b	b	b	4
	48207538	03/99/99	b	b	b	b	b	X	X	X	b	X	b	b	b	X	b	b	b	5
	48207541	04/99/99	b	b	b	b	b	X	X	X	b	X	b	b	b	X	b	b	b	5
	48207544	05/99/99	b	b	b	b	b	X	X	X	b	X	b	b	b	X	b	b	b	5
	48207547	02/99/99	b	b	b	b	b	X	X	X	b	X	b	b	b	X	b	b	b	5
	48207550	06/99/99	b	b	b	b	b	X	X	X	b	X	b	b	b	X	b	b	b	5
	48207553	99/01/99	b	b	b	b	b	X	X	X	b	X	b	b	b	b	b	b	b	4
	48207556	01/99/99	b	b	b	b	b	b	b	b	b	b	b	b	b	b	b	b	b	0
	48207559	03/99/99	b	b	b	b	b	b	b	b	b	b	b	b	b	b	b	b	b	0

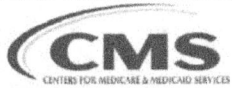

MDS 3.0 Resident Level Quality Measure Report

Facility ID: ▓▓▓▓▓

Facility Name: ▓▓▓▓▓

CCN: ▓▓▓▓▓

City/State: ▓▓▓▓▓

Report Period: 04/01/2021 - 09/30/2021

Report Run Date: 10/07/2021

Data Calculation Date: 10/04/2021

Report Version Number: 3.03

Note: S = short stay, L = long stay; X = triggered, b = not triggered or excluded,
C = complete; data available for all days selected, I = incomplete; data not available for all days selected

Resident Name	Resident ID	Admission Date	Discharge Date	Pressure Ulcer/Injury[1]
▓▓▓▓▓	48203481	01/05/2021	01/12/2021	b
▓▓▓▓▓	48204570	08/12/2021	08/19/2021	b
▓▓▓▓▓	48204852	11/23/2020	11/30/2020	b
▓▓▓▓▓	48205443	08/25/2021	09/01/2021	b
▓▓▓▓▓	48966432	01/05/2021	01/12/2021	b
▓▓▓▓▓	48967513	11/23/2020	11/30/2020	b
▓▓▓▓▓	48207689	04/23/2021	04/30/2021	b
▓▓▓▓▓	48200303	01/08/2021	01/15/2021	b
▓▓▓▓▓	48207789	08/11/2021	08/18/2021	X
▓▓▓▓▓	48965807	01/08/2021	01/15/2021	b
▓▓▓▓▓	48203482	01/06/2021	01/13/2021	b
▓▓▓▓▓	48204571	08/13/2021	08/20/2021	b
▓▓▓▓▓	48204853	11/24/2020	12/01/2020	b
▓▓▓▓▓	48205444	08/26/2021	09/02/2021	b

[1] The Changes in Skin Integrity Post-Acute Care: Pressure Ulcer/Injury (S038.02) measure is calculated using the SNF QRP measure specifications v3.0 addendum and is based on 12 months of data (10/01/2020 - 09/30/2021).

27

Monthly comparison report

The monthly comparison report summarizes the nursing facility's performance with the averages for the state and the nation. It's an easy way to compare observed and adjusted percentages for each quality measure for a specified 6-month period.

Public data: Because the monthly comparison report is intended for public use, data with small denominators or high-triggered percentages are suppressed. Small denominators are defined as <30 for long-stay measures and <20 for short-stay measures.

Frequency of calculation: The monthly comparison report data are calculated on the first day of each month, with assessment data from two months prior.

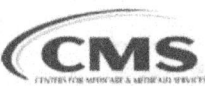

Facility ID: ▓▓▓▓▓
CCN: ▓▓▓▓
Facility Name: ▓▓▓▓▓▓▓
City/State: ▓▓▓▓▓▓

Report Period: 04/01/2021 - 09/30/2021
Report Run Date: 10/01/2021
Data Calculation Date: 10/04/2021
Report Version Number: 3.03

Note: S = short stay, L = long stay
Note: C = complete; data available for all days selected, I = incomplete; data not available for all days selected
Note: N/A represents a value that could not be computed

Long Stay Measure (Sample size = 53)
Short Stay Measure (Sample size = 1348)

CMS ID	Data	Measure Description	Facility Percent	State Percent	National Percent
N015.03	C	Hi-risk/Unstageable Pres Ulcer (L)	6.8%	6.8%	6.8%
N027.02	C	Phys restraints (L)	1.7%	1.7%	1.7%
N032.02	C	Falls (L)	5.6%	5.6%	5.6%
N013.02	C	Falls w/Maj Injury (L)	3.7%	3.7%	3.7%
N011.02	C	Antipsych Med (S)	>=90%	91.3%	91.3%
N031.03	C	Antipsych Med (L)	>=90%	99.7%	99.7%
N033.02	C	Antianxiety/Hypnotic Prev (L)	>=90%	99.7%	99.7%
N036.02	C	Antianxiety/Hypnotic % (L)	>=90%	99.7%	99.7%
N034.02	C	Behav Sx affect Others (L)	0.0%	0.0%	0.0%
N030.02	C	Depress Sx (L)	>=90%	100.0%	100.0%
N024.02	C	UTI (L)	0.6%	0.6%	0.6%
N026.03	C	Cath Insert/Left Bladder (L)	14.0%	14.0%	14.0%
N025.02	C	Lo-Risk Lose B/B Con (L)	0.0%	0.0%	0.0%
N029.02	C	Excess Wt Loss (L)	>=90%	98.8%	98.8%
N028.02	C	Incr ADL Help (L)	17.2%	17.2%	17.2%
N035.03	C	Move Indep Worsens (L)	40.1%	40.1%	40.1%
N037.03	C	Improvement in Function (S)	>=90%	100.0%	100.0%
S038.02	C	Pressure Ulcer/Injury[1]	1.8%	N/A	0.6%

[1] The Changes in Skin Integrity Post-Acute Care: Pressure Ulcer/Injury (S038.02) measure is calculated using the SNF QRP measure specifications v3.0 addendum and is based on 12 months of data (10/01/2020 - 09/30/2021).

Chapter 3: Common terms and definitions

Some sections of the resident assessment instrument (RAI) have MDS elements that affect the calculations of quality measures. Here are some of the trickier ones to get right.

- **D**: Mood
- **E**: Behavior
- **G**: Functional status
- **H**: Bladder and bowel
- **I**: Active diagnoses
- **J**: Health conditions
- **K**: Swallowing and nutritional status
- **M**: Skin conditions
- **N**: Medications
- **O**: Special treatments, procedures, and programs
- **P**: Restraints and alarms
- **V**: Care area assessment (CAA) summary
- **X**: Correction request
- **Z**: Assessment administration

Here are some common terms and their definitions:

Episode: a period of time spanning one or more stays

Short-stay resident: a resident who has been in the nursing home for 100 days or fewer.

Long-stay resident: a resident who has been in the nursing home for more than 100 days.

Risk adjustment: "Our patients are sicker" is a commonly heard whine in healthcare. But it's true, facilities with higher numbers of sicker patients or patients who have more comorbidities will have artificially lower quality scores. Risk adjustment levels the playing field. Facilities with high numbers of covariates have their scores improved to the levels of facilities with low numbers of covariates.

Covariate: Quality measures are risk adjusted using resident-level covariates. Covariates have a value of 1 if the condition is present and 0 if the condition is not present.

Lookback scan: The lookback period is the length of a resident's entire Medicare Part A SNF stay.

Section D (mood)

Percent of residents who have depressive symptoms (long stay)

This quality measure reports the percentage of long-stay residents who have had symptoms of depression during the 2-week period before the MDS target date.

Lookback period: 14 days

Data source: resident mood interview or staff assessment of mood

The percent of residents who have depressive symptoms (long stay) is a quality measure that measures the presence of two specific symptoms of depression. The resident has to have the symptoms at least half of the time during the lookback period.

The two symptoms are:

- little interest or pleasure in doing things
- feeling or appearing down, depressed, or hopeless

D0200: Resident Mood Interview (PHQ-9©)

D0200. Resident Mood Interview (PHQ-9©)

Say to resident: *"Over the last 2 weeks, have you been bothered by any of the following problems?"*

If symptom is present, enter 1 (yes) in column 1, Symptom Presence.
If yes in column 1, then ask the resident: *"About **how often** have you been bothered by this?"*
Read and show the resident a card with the symptom frequency choices. Indicate response in column 2, Symptom Frequency.

1. Symptom Presence	2. Symptom Frequency		
0. **No** (enter 0 in column 2) 1. **Yes** (enter 0-3 in column 2) 9. **No response** (leave column 2 blank)	0. **Never or 1 day** 1. **2-6 days** (several days) 2. **7-11 days** (half or more of the days) 3. **12-14 days** (nearly every day)	**1.** Symptom Presence	**2.** Symptom Frequency
		↓ Enter Scores in Boxes ↓	
A. *Little interest or pleasure in doing things*		☐	☐
B. *Feeling down, depressed, or hopeless*		☐	☐
C. *Trouble falling or staying asleep, or sleeping too much*		☐	☐
D. *Feeling tired or having little energy*		☐	☐
E. *Poor appetite or overeating*		☐	☐
F. *Feeling bad about yourself - or that you are a failure or have let yourself or your family down*		☐	☐
G. *Trouble concentrating on things, such as reading the newspaper or watching television*		☐	☐
H. *Moving or speaking so slowly that other people could have noticed. Or the opposite - being so fidgety or restless that you have been moving around a lot more than usual*		☐	☐
I. *Thoughts that you would be better off dead, or of hurting yourself in some way*		☐	☐

If the long-stay resident did the **resident mood interview**, they must meet both condition A1 and condition B1:

Condition A1:

- **D0200-A2** (little interest or pleasure in doing things)
    - **2** (7-11 days) or **3** (12-14 days)

or

- **D0200-B2** (feeling down, depressed, or hopeless)
    - **2** (7-11 days) or **3** (12-14 days)

D0300: Total Severity Score

D0300. Total Severity Score	
Enter Score ☐☐	**Add scores for all frequency responses in Column 2,** Symptom Frequency. Total score must be between 00 and 27. Enter 99 if unable to complete interview (i.e., Symptom Frequency is blank for 3 or more items).

Condition B1:

The resident interview total severity score indicates the presence of depression. This means that D0300 $\geq$ 10 and $\leq$ 27.

If the long-stay resident did the **staff assessment of resident mood**, they must meet both condition A2 and condition B2:

Condition A2:

- **D0500-A2** (little interest or pleasure in doing things)
    - **2** (7-11 days) or **3** (12-14 days)

or

- **D0500-B2** (feeling tired or having little energy)
    - **2** (7-11 days) or **3** (12-14 days)

D0600. Total Severity Score	
Enter Score	**Add scores for all frequency responses in Column 2,** Symptom Frequency. Total score must be between 00 and 30.

Condition B2:

The staff assessment total severity score indicates the presence of depression. This means that D0600 $\geq$ 10 and $\leq$ 47.

Tricky parts

This quality measure uses these two items from the PHQ-9 or the PHQ-9-OV:

- little interest or pleasure in doing things
- feeling down, depressed, or hopeless

It's important that all the staff know how to ask questions and get accurate answers. They should be trained to observe all symptoms, even if they don't think it relates to depression. Assessors should also interview staff from the shifts that know the resident knows best.

If the staff can't get answers from the resident or don't attempt the interview, they may have to code dashes. Frequent dashes can skew the score of this quality measure.

D0500: Staff Assessment of Resident Mood (PHQ-9-OV©)

D0500. Staff Assessment of Resident Mood (PHQ-9-OV*)	1. Symptom Presence	2. Symptom Frequency
Do not conduct if Resident Mood Interview (D0200-D0300) was completed		
Over the last 2 weeks, did the resident have any of the following problems or behaviors?		
If symptom is present, enter 1 (yes) in column 1, Symptom Presence. Then move to column 2, Symptom Frequency, and indicate symptom frequency.		
1. Symptom Presence 0. **No** (enter 0 in column 2) 1. **Yes** (enter 0-3 in column 2) **2. Symptom Frequency** 0. **Never or 1 day** 1. **2-6 days** (several days) 2. **7-11 days** (half or more of the days) 3. **12-14 days** (nearly every day)	↓ Enter Scores in Boxes ↓	
A. Little interest or pleasure in doing things	☐	☐
B. Feeling or appearing down, depressed, or hopeless	☐	☐
C. Trouble falling or staying asleep, or sleeping too much	☐	☐
D. Feeling tired or having little energy	☐	☐
E. Poor appetite or overeating	☐	☐
F. Indicating that s/he feels bad about self, is a failure, or has let self or family down	☐	☐
G. Trouble concentrating on things, such as reading the newspaper or watching television	☐	☐
H. Moving or speaking so slowly that other people have noticed. Or the opposite - being so fidgety or restless that s/he has been moving around a lot more than usual	☐	☐
I. States that life isn't worth living, wishes for death, or attempts to harm self	☐	☐
J. Being short-tempered, easily annoyed	☐	☐

Section E (behavior)

Prevalence of behavior symptoms affecting others (long stay)

This quality measure identifies all the residents who have behavioral symptoms, rejection of care, and wandering.

Lookback period: 7 days

Data source:

- **E0200-A** (physical behavioral symptoms directed toward others)
- **E200-B** (verbal behavioral symptoms directed toward others)
- **E0200-C** (other behavioral symptoms directed toward others)
- **E0800** (rejection of care)
- **E0900** (wandering)

E0200: Behavioral Symptom—Presence & Frequency

E0200. Behavioral Symptom - Presence & Frequency		
Note presence of symptoms and their frequency		
	↓ Enter Codes in Boxes	
Coding: 0. **Behavior not exhibited** 1. **Behavior of this type occurred 1 to 3 days** 2. **Behavior of this type occurred 4 to 6 days,** but less than daily 3. **Behavior of this type occurred daily**	☐	**A.** **Physical behavioral symptoms directed toward others** (e.g., hitting, kicking, pushing, scratching, grabbing, abusing others sexually)
	☐	**B.** **Verbal behavioral symptoms directed toward others** (e.g., threatening others, screaming at others, cursing at others)
	☐	**C.** **Other behavioral symptoms not directed toward others** (e.g., physical symptoms such as hitting or scratching self, pacing, rummaging, public sexual acts, disrobing in public, throwing or smearing food or bodily wastes, or verbal/vocal symptoms like screaming, disruptive sounds)

E0800: Rejection of Care—Presence & Frequency

E0800. Rejection of Care - Presence & Frequency	
Enter Code ☐	**Did the resident reject evaluation or care** (e.g., bloodwork, taking medications, ADL assistance) **that is necessary to achieve the resident's goals for health and well-being?** Do not include behaviors that have already been addressed (e.g., by discussion or care planning with the resident or family), and determined to be consistent with resident values, preferences, or goals. 0. **Behavior not exhibited** 1. **Behavior of this type occurred 1 to 3 days** 2. **Behavior of this type occurred 4 to 6 days,** but less than daily 3. **Behavior of this type occurred daily**

E0900: Wandering—Presence & Frequency

E0900. Wandering - Presence & Frequency	
Enter Code ☐	**Has the resident wandered?** 0. **Behavior not exhibited** ➝ Skip to E1100, Change in Behavior or Other Symptoms 1. **Behavior of this type occurred 1 to 3 days** 2. **Behavior of this type occurred 4 to 6 days**, but less than daily 3. **Behavior of this type occurred daily**

Calculations

This measure consists of long-stay residents who have any of the 5 items coded 1, 2, or 3, meaning that the behavioral occurred at least once.

- **E0200-A** (physical behavioral symptoms directed toward others) = 1, 2, or 3
- **E200-B** (verbal behavioral symptoms directed toward others) = 1, 2, or 3
- **E0200-C** (other behavioral symptoms directed toward others) = 1, 2, or 3
- **E0800** (rejection of care) = 1, 2, or 3
- **E0900** (wandering) = 1, 2, or 3

Tricky parts

This quality measure doesn't use items E0500 (impact on resident) or E600 (impact on others). But if the other 5 items occurred even once, the resident is counted in the quality measure. So, it's important for staff members to understand the definitions of each behavior.

Section G (functional status)

Percent of residents who made improvements in function (short stay)

This quality measure is the percent of short-stay residents who made improvements in their function. This means that between admission and discharge, they have gained more independence in transfers, locomotion, and walking.

The residents' function is measured with the **mid-loss activities of daily living** (**MLADL**) score. A negative MLADL change in score means an improvement in function, because lower numbers mean more independence. The MLADL score is the sum of:

- **G0110-B1**: transfer (self-performance)
- **G0110-D1**: walk in corridor (self-performance)
- **G0110-E1**: locomotion on unit (self-performance)

G0110: Activities of Daily Living (ADL) Assistance

G0110. Activities of Daily Living (ADL) Assistance
Refer to the ADL flow chart in the RAI manual to facilitate accurate coding

Instructions for Rule of 3
- When an activity occurs three times at any one given level, code that level.
- When an activity occurs three times at multiple levels, code the most dependent, exceptions are total dependence (4), activity must require full assist every time, and activity did not occur (8), activity must not have occurred at all. Example, three times extensive assistance (3) and three times limited assistance (2), code extensive assistance (3).
- When an activity occurs at various levels, but not three times at any given level, apply the following:
  - When there is a combination of full staff performance, and extensive assistance, code extensive assistance.
  - When there is a combination of full staff performance, weight bearing assistance and/or non-weight bearing assistance code limited assistance (2).

If none of the above are met, code supervision.

1. **ADL Self-Performance**
   Code for **resident's performance** over all shifts - not including setup. If the ADL activity occurred 3 or more times at various levels of assistance, code the most dependent - except for total dependence, which requires full staff performance every time

   Coding:

   Activity Occurred 3 or More Times
   0. **Independent** - no help or staff oversight at any time
   1. **Supervision** - oversight, encouragement or cueing
   2. **Limited assistance** - resident highly involved in activity; staff provide guided maneuvering of limbs or other non-weight-bearing assistance
   3. **Extensive assistance** - resident involved in activity, staff provide weight-bearing support
   4. **Total dependence** - full staff performance every time during entire 7-day period

   Activity Occurred 2 or Fewer Times
   7. **Activity occurred only once or twice** - activity did occur but only once or twice
   8. **Activity did not occur** - activity did not occur or family and/or non-facility staff provided care 100% of the time for that activity over the entire 7-day period

2. **ADL Support Provided**
   Code for **most support provided** over all shifts; code regardless of resident's self-performance classification

   Coding:
   0. **No** setup or physical help from staff
   1. **Setup** help only
   2. **One** person physical assist
   3. **Two+** persons physical assist
   8. ADL activity itself **did not occur** or family and/or non-facility staff provided care 100% of the time for that activity over the entire 7-day period

	1. Self-Performance	2. Support
	↓ Enter Codes in Boxes ↓	
A. **Bed mobility** - how resident moves to and from lying position, turns side to side, and positions body while in bed or alternate sleep furniture	☐	☐
B. **Transfer** - how resident moves between surfaces including to or from: bed, chair, wheelchair, standing position (**excludes** to/from bath/toilet)	☐	☐
C. **Walk in room** - how resident walks between locations in his/her room	☐	☐
D. **Walk in corridor** - how resident walks in corridor on unit	☐	☐
E. **Locomotion on unit** - how resident moves between locations in his/her room and adjacent corridor on same floor. If in wheelchair, self-sufficiency once in chair	☐	☐
F. **Locomotion off unit** - how resident moves to and returns from off-unit locations (e.g., areas set aside for dining, activities or treatments). **If facility has only one floor**, how resident moves to and from distant areas on the floor. If in wheelchair, self-sufficiency once in chair	☐	☐
G. **Dressing** - how resident puts on, fastens and takes off all items of clothing, including donning/removing a prosthesis or TED hose. Dressing includes putting on and changing pajamas and housedresses	☐	☐
H. **Eating** - how resident eats and drinks, regardless of skill. Do not include eating/drinking during medication pass. Includes intake of nourishment by other means (e.g., tube feeding, total parenteral nutrition, IV fluids administered for nutrition or hydration)	☐	☐
I. **Toilet use** - how resident uses the toilet room, commode, bedpan, or urinal; transfers on/off toilet; cleanses self after elimination; changes pad; manages ostomy or catheter; and adjusts clothes. Do not include emptying of bedpan, urinal, bedside commode, catheter bag or ostomy bag	☐	☐
J. **Personal hygiene** - how resident maintains personal hygiene, including combing hair, brushing teeth, shaving, applying makeup, washing/drying face and hands (**excludes** baths and showers)	☐	☐

Short-stay residents are defined as people who spend 100 or fewer days cumulatively in a nursing facility. The calculation uses the time period from the earliest initial assessment to the discharge assessment.

> **Valid initial assessments**: The short stay resident should have either a 5-day assessment or an admission assessment. If a resident has both a 5-day assessment and an admission assessment, then the earlier one is the considered the earliest assessment. So, the earliest date is what's used in the calculation for the quality measure.

> **Discharge assessment**: The discharge assessment is item A0310-F = 10, which means that it's a discharge assessment with no anticipated return to nursing home.

A0310.	Type of Assessment

Enter Code [ ][ ]	A. **Federal OBRA Reason for Assessment** 01. **Admission** assessment (required by day 14) 02. **Quarterly** review assessment 03. **Annual** assessment 04. **Significant change in status** assessment 05. **Significant correction** to **prior comprehensive** assessment 06. **Significant correction** to **prior quarterly** assessment 99. **None of the above**
Enter Code [ ][ ]	B. **PPS Assessment** **PPS Scheduled Assessment for a Medicare Part A Stay** 01. **5-day** scheduled assessment **PPS Unscheduled Assessment for a Medicare Part A Stay** 08. **IPA** - Interim Payment Assessment **Not PPS Assessment** 99. **None of the above**
Enter Code [ ]	E. **Is this assessment the first assessment** (OBRA, Scheduled PPS, or Discharge) **since the most recent admission/entry or reentry?** 0. **No** 1. **Yes**
Enter Code [ ][ ]	F. **Entry/discharge reporting** 01. **Entry** tracking record 10. **Discharge** assessment-**return not anticipated** 11. **Discharge** assessment-**return anticipated** 12. **Death in facility** tracking record 99. **None of the above**
Enter Code [ ]	G. **Type of discharge** - Complete only if A0310F = 10 or 11 1. **Planned** 2. **Unplanned**
Enter Code [ ]	G1. **Is this a SNF Part A Interrupted Stay?** 0. **No** 1. **Yes**
Enter Code [ ]	H. **Is this a SNF Part A PPS Discharge Assessment?** 0. **No** 1. **Yes**

Mid-loss of activities daily living (MLADL) performance score

This quality measure only includes residents who have a negative change in their mid-loss of activities daily living (MLADL) performance score. You compare the score on the discharge date to the 5-day or the admission assessment date, whichever is earlier. The sum of the MLADLs on the discharge date must be less than the initial assessment date.

The performance score is calculated as the sum of:

- **G0110-B1**: transfer (self-performance)
- **G0110-D1**: walk in corridor (self-performance)
- **G0110-E1**: locomotion on unit (self-performance)

If a resident got a score of 7 (activity occurred only once or twice) or 8 (activity did not occur), then it will be recoded to 4 (total dependence) for these calculations.

Tricky parts: MLADL scores

The accuracy of this quality metric and the MLADL score depends on the accuracy of section G0110's activities of daily living (ADL) scoring. Section G is notoriously difficult to code to begin with, so this is no small feat. For example, G0110-E (locomotion) can be tricky because it refers to how the resident moves in both his room and in the adjacent corridor. If this occurred at least 3 times in the last 7 days, then the assessor has to code the highest level of assistance that the resident needed. The coder should talk to the staff or a family member who interacted with the resident during the lookback period to get the most accurate answer.

Covariates – our patients are sicker

A covariate is something that increases the risk of an outcome. If there were no covariate factor, facilities with large number of residents with covariate conditions would have higher scores than facilities with a small number of residents with covariate conditions.

This measure's covariates are:

> **A0900**: age (≤ 54, 55–84, or > 84)

> **A0800**: gender

> **C0500**, **C0700**, and **C1000**: severe cognitive impairment (

> **G0110-A1**, **G0110-B1**, **G0110-E1**, **G0110-G1**, **G0110-H1**, **G0110-I1**, **G0110-J1**: long-form ADL scale, categorized by tercile in the quarter

> **I0600**: heart failure

> **I4500**: CVA, TIA, or stroke

> **I3900**: hip fracture

> **I4000**: other fracture

Tricky parts: covariates

Lookback period: 7 days

The data for covariates is from section I (active diagnoses), so the staff have to code that section correctly. A resident can get an active diagnosis in several ways:

- A physician, nurse practitioner, physician assistant, or clinical nurse specialist diagnoses the resident
- The diagnosis had a direct affect on the resident's functional status, cognitive status, mood or behavior, medical treatments, nursing monitoring, or risk of death during the 7-day lookback period
- Clinical evidence of the problem during the 7-day lookback period

Tricky parts: comparison percentile groups

This metric is tricky because it's reported positively, while most other nursing home metrics report negatively. Let's say that your percent of residents who made improvements in function is positive. Good job. But because the metric is reported opposite, the comparison group national percentile is also opposite. With most measures, a 75th percentile or higher automatically puts you under review. With percent of residents who made improvements in function, a 25th percentile or lower automatically puts you under review.

Percent of residents whose need for help with activities of daily living has increased (long stay)

This quality measure is percent of long-stay residents whose need for help with late-loss activities of daily living (ADLs) has increased when compared to the prior assessment.

An increase is defined as an increase of 2 or more coding points in one late loss ADL item or an increase of 1 coding point in two or more late loss ADL items.

Data sources: The four late-loss ADL items are:

- **G0110-A1**: bed mobility (self-performance)
- **G0110-B1**: transfer (self-performance)
- **G0110-H1**: eating (self-performance)
- **G0110-I1**: toileting (self-performance)

You calculate the late-loss activities of daily living by subtracting the most recent late loss ADL score from the prior late loss ADL score. The most recent assessment is also called the **target assessment**. The assessment that came before the target assessment is the **prior assessment**.

A resident is classified as having an increased need of help with late-loss ADLs if they meet either condition A or condition B.

> Note: Same as the mid-loss score, if a resident got a score of 7 (activity occurred only once or twice) or 8 (activity did not occur), then it will be recoded to 4 (total dependence) for these calculations.

Condition A, two level decline in one area

Under condition A, the resident increased 2 or more points in one ADL item.

At least **one** of the following must be true:

1. Bed mobility at target assessment at least 2 points higher than at prior assessment

   G0110-A1 (bed mobility) – G0110-A1 (bed mobility) ≥ 2
   target assessment   prior assessment

2. Transfer at target assessment at least 2 points higher than at prior assessment

   G0110-B1 (transfer) – G0110-B1 (transfer) ≥ 2
   target assessment   prior assessment

3. Eating at target assessment at least 2 points higher than at prior assessment

   G0110-H1 (eating) – G0110-H1 (eating) ≥ 2
   target assessment   prior assessment

4. Toileting at target assessment at least 2 points higher than at prior assessment

   G0110-I1 (toileting) – G0110-I1 (toileting) ≥ 2
   target assessment   prior assessment

Condition B, one level decline in two or more areas

Under condition B, the resident increased 1 point in two or more ADL items.

At least **two** of the following must be true:

1. Bed mobility at target assessment at least 1 point higher than at prior assessment

   G0110-A1 (bed mobility) – G0110-A1 (bed mobility) $\geq$ 1
   _{target assessment}   _{prior assessment}

2. Transfer at target assessment at least 1 point higher than at prior assessment

   G0110-B1 (transfer) – G0110-B1 (transfer) $\geq$ 1
   _{target assessment}   _{prior assessment}

3. Eating at target assessment at least 1 point higher than at prior assessment

   G0110-H1 (eating) – G0110-H1 (eating) $\geq$ 1
   _{target assessment}   _{prior assessment}

4. Toileting at target assessment at least 1 point higher than at prior assessment

   G0110-I1 (toileting) – G0110-I1 (toileting) $\geq$ 1
   _{target assessment}   _{prior assessment}

Percent of residents whose ability to move independently worsened (long stay)

This quality measure shows the percentage of long-stay residents whose ability to move independently worsened, or who experienced a decline in independence of locomotion.

> Long-stay residents are defined as people who have stayed at the nursing home for more than 100 days.

Data sources: A decline is considered an increase of 1 or more points on the G0100E, comparing the target assessment to the prior assessment.

- G0110-E1 (locomotion on unit)

Period of time: You compare the decline of the most recent resident assessment to the assessment before that one. The most recent assessment is the target assessment and the one before that one is the prior assessment.

Calculation for loss of locomotion

Decline is an increase of at least one point in locomotion on unit, self-performance, from the prior assessment to the target assessment. The formula for identifying decline is:

$$\text{G0110-E1} \left(\substack{\text{locomotion on unit,} \\ \text{self performance}} \right) - \text{G0110-E1} \left(\substack{\text{locomotion on unit,} \\ \text{self performance}} \right) \geq 1$$

target assessment   prior assessment

If a resident got a score of 7 (activity occurred only once or twice) or 8 (activity did not occur), then it will be recoded to 4 (total dependence) for these calculations.

Covariates

Most of the covariates are from section G (functional issues) or section C (cognitive patterns).

- **G0110-H1** (eating, self-performance): needs help, dependence
- **G0110-I1** (toilet use, self-performance): needs help, dependence
- **G0110-B1** (transfer, self-performance): needs help, dependence
- **G0110-D1** (walking in corridor, self-performance): independence, needs some help, needs more help
- **C0500**, **C0700**, and **C1000** (severe cognitive impairment)
- **A0900** (linear age)
- **A0800** (gender)
- **B1000** (vision change score): a positive change in score from prior assessment to latest assessment)
- **O0100-C2** (oxygen use): no oxygen use on prior assessment and latest assessment

Tricky parts

The definition of G0110-E (locomotion on unit) is how the resident moves between locations in his room and adjacent corridors on the same floor. Sometimes people think G0110-E only means locomotion in the resident's bedroom. It's important for staff to observe how the resident moves in the hallways and common rooms too.

Section H (bladder and bowel)

Percent of low-risk residents who lose control of their bowel or bladder (long stay)

Reporting period: 90 days

This quality measure identifies low-risk, long-stay residents who lose control of their bowel or bladder. This means residents who are frequently or always incontinent.

Risk for incontinence: Cognitive impairment and ADL dependency can lead to incontinence, but it's more unusual for those without those conditions to be incontinent. If this quality measure is high, then the nursing home should re-evaluate their system for managing incontinence. High-risk residents are defined as those with severe cognitive impairment, or total dependence in bed mobility, transfer, or locomotion self-performance.

Data source: The MDS items that this quality measure uses are:

- **H0300** (urinary continence)
- **H0400** (bowel continence)

Calculations

Residents with the following items are frequently or always incontinent.

- H0300 (urinary continence) = 2 or 3
- H0400 (bowel continence) = 2 or 3

H0300. Urinary Continence	
Enter Code	**Urinary continence -** Select the one category that best describes the resident 0. **Always continent** 1. **Occasionally incontinent** (less than 7 episodes of incontinence) 2. **Frequently incontinent** (7 or more episodes of urinary incontinence, but at least one episode of continent voiding) 3. **Always incontinent** (no episodes of continent voiding) 9. **Not rated,** resident had a catheter (indwelling, condom), urinary ostomy, or no urine output for the entire 7 days

H0400. Bowel Continence	
Enter Code	**Bowel continence -** Select the one category that best describes the resident 0. **Always continent** 1. **Occasionally incontinent** (one episode of bowel incontinence) 2. **Frequently incontinent** (2 or more episodes of bowel incontinence, but at least one continent bowel movement) 3. **Always incontinent** (no episodes of continent bowel movements) 9. **Not rated,** resident had an ostomy or did not have a bowel movement for the entire 7 days

Tricky parts

Staff should document episodes of incontinence, instead of a single entry per shift. Otherwise, it's easy to miss residents who are frequently incontinent.

Percent of residents who had a catheter inserted and left in their bladder (long stay)

This quality measure shows the percentage of long-stay residents who indwelling catheters or catheters inserted and left in their bladder.

> Long-stay residents are defined as people who have stayed at the nursing home for more than 100 days.

The reporting period is 90 days. The admission and 5-day assessments are not included in the reporting period.

H0100. Appliances	
↓ Check all that apply	
☐	A. **Indwelling catheter** (including suprapubic catheter and nephrostomy tube)
☐	B. **External catheter**
☐	C. **Ostomy** (including urostomy, ileostomy, and colostomy)
☐	D. **Intermittent catheterization**
☐	Z. **None of the above**

Data source:

- **H0100-A** (indwelling catheter)

Long-stay residents with a selected target assessment that indicates the use of indwelling catheters (H0100A = [1])

Covariates

Covariates adjust for facilities with a larger number of residents with conditions that can affect quality measures. This quality measure adjusts for:

- Residents who had incontinence before admission to the nursing home or before their first assessment
- Pressure ulcers, stage 2, 3, or 4

Tricky parts

A common pitfall is a missing diagnosis on the MDS in section I. Additionally, it may be worthwhile to review residents with either a cerebral or spinal diagnosis, such as cerebrovascular accident (CVA), multiple sclerosis (MS), or stenosis, as they may have a neurogenic bladder but are missing the diagnosis in section I. Also, review residents with benign prostatic hyperplasia (BPH) and/or prostate or bladder cancer, as they may have obstructive uropathy but, again, are missing the diagnosis.

Section I (active diagnoses)

Percent of residents with a urinary tract infection (long stay)

Reporting period: 30 days

This quality measure is the percentage of long-stay residents who had a urinary tract infection on their last assessment.

Tricky parts

This quality measure can be inaccurate due to over-coding, which results in a higher percentage than it should be. Sometimes people will check I2300 (urinary tract infection (UTI) within the last 30 days) only because a physician diagnosed the resident with a UTI and started treatment. But actually, you should only code UTI on the MDS if both of these two requirements are met:

1. Resident is diagnosed with an evidence-based criterion such as McGeer, NHSN, or Loeb
2. A physician must have documented the UTI. Some states allow a nurse practitioner, physician assistant, or clinical nurse specialist to also do this

I: Active Diagnoses in the Last 7 Days

Active Diagnoses in the last 7 days - Check all that apply
Diagnoses listed in parentheses are provided as examples and should not be considered as all-inclusive lists

Cancer
- [ ] I0100. Cancer (with or without metastasis)

Heart/Circulation
- [ ] I0200. Anemia (e.g., aplastic, iron deficiency, pernicious, and sickle cell)
- [ ] I0300. Atrial Fibrillation or Other Dysrhythmias (e.g., bradycardias and tachycardias)
- [ ] I0400. Coronary Artery Disease (CAD) (e.g., angina, myocardial infarction, and atherosclerotic heart disease (ASHD))
- [ ] I0500. Deep Venous Thrombosis (DVT), Pulmonary Embolus (PE), or Pulmonary Thrombo-Embolism (PTE)
- [ ] I0600. Heart Failure (e.g., congestive heart failure (CHF) and pulmonary edema)
- [ ] I0700. Hypertension
- [ ] I0800. Orthostatic Hypotension
- [ ] I0900. Peripheral Vascular Disease (PVD) or Peripheral Arterial Disease (PAD)

Gastrointestinal
- [ ] I1100. Cirrhosis
- [ ] I1200. Gastroesophageal Reflux Disease (GERD) or Ulcer (e.g., esophageal, gastric, and peptic ulcers)
- [ ] I1300. Ulcerative Colitis, Crohn's Disease, or Inflammatory Bowel Disease

Genitourinary
- [ ] I1400. Benign Prostatic Hyperplasia (BPH)
- [ ] I1500. Renal Insufficiency, Renal Failure, or End-Stage Renal Disease (ESRD)
- [ ] I1550. Neurogenic Bladder
- [ ] I1650. Obstructive Uropathy

Infections
- [ ] I1700. Multidrug-Resistant Organism (MDRO)
- [ ] I2000. Pneumonia
- [ ] I2100. Septicemia
- [ ] I2200. Tuberculosis
- [ ] I2300. Urinary Tract Infection (UTI) (LAST 30 DAYS)
- [ ] I2400. Viral Hepatitis (e.g., Hepatitis A, B, C, D, and E)
- [ ] I2500. Wound Infection (other than foot)

Metabolic
- [ ] I2900. Diabetes Mellitus (DM) (e.g., diabetic retinopathy, nephropathy, and neuropathy)
- [ ] I3100. Hyponatremia
- [ ] I3200. Hyperkalemia
- [ ] I3300. Hyperlipidemia (e.g., hypercholesterolemia)
- [ ] I3400. Thyroid Disorder (e.g., hypothyroidism, hyperthyroidism, and Hashimoto's thyroiditis)

Musculoskeletal
- [ ] I3700. Arthritis (e.g., degenerative joint disease (DJD), osteoarthritis, and rheumatoid arthritis (RA))
- [ ] I3800. Osteoporosis
- [ ] I3900. Hip Fracture - any hip fracture that has a relationship to current status, treatments, monitoring (e.g., sub-capital fractures, and fractures of the trochanter and femoral neck)
- [ ] I4000. Other Fracture

Neurological
- [ ] I4200. Alzheimer's Disease
- [ ] I4300. Aphasia
- [ ] I4400. Cerebral Palsy
- [ ] I4500. Cerebrovascular Accident (CVA), Transient Ischemic Attack (TIA), or Stroke
- [ ] I4800. Non-Alzheimer's Dementia (e.g. Lewy body dementia, vascular or multi-infarct dementia; mixed dementia; frontotemporal dementia such as Pick's disease; and dementia related to stroke, Parkinson's or Creutzfeldt-Jakob diseases)

Neurological Diagnoses continued on next page

Section J (health conditions)

Prevalence of falls (long stay)

Lookback scan: 275 days

This quality measure is the percentage of long-stay residents who fell in the lookback scan.

Data source:

- **J1800**

J1800. Any Falls Since Admission/Entry or Reentry or Prior Assessment (OBRA or Scheduled PPS), whichever is more recent	
Enter Code	Has the resident **had any falls since admission/entry or reentry or the prior assessment** (OBRA or Scheduled PPS), whichever is more recent?
	0. **No** → Skip to J2000, Prior Surgery
	1. **Yes** → Continue to J1900, Number of Falls Since Admission/Entry or Reentry or Prior Assessment (OBRA or Scheduled PPS)

If J1800 = 1, then the resident is counted as having a fall.

Tricky parts

This quality measure looks at falls that occurred during look-back scan, with a target date going back 275 days. So, it uses information not just from the most recent assessment, but in the last three months.

Percent of residents experiencing one or more falls with major injury (long stay)

This quality measure is the percentage of long-stay residents who had at least one fall that resulted in a major injury. Examples of major injuries are bone fractures, joint dislocations, closed head injuries with altered consciousness, and subdural hematomas.

Data source:

- ## J1900-C

J1900. Number of Falls Since Admission/Entry or Reentry or Prior Assessment (OBRA or Scheduled PPS), whichever is more recent		
	↓ **Enter Codes in Boxes**	
Coding: 0. **None** 1. **One** 2. **Two or more**	☐	**A. No injury** - no evidence of any injury is noted on physical assessment by the nurse or primary care clinician; no complaints of pain or injury by the resident; no change in the resident's behavior is noted after the fall
	☐	**B. Injury (except major)** - skin tears, abrasions, lacerations, superficial bruises, hematomas and sprains; or any fall-related injury that causes the resident to complain of pain
	☐	**C. Major injury** - bone fractures, joint dislocations, closed head injuries with altered consciousness, subdural hematoma

If J1900-C = 1 or 2, then then the resident is counted as having a fall with a major injury.

Tricky parts

The time period for this qualifying measure lasts one episode or lookback scan, which may span more than one stay. Additionally, the MDS definition of a major injury may not match your state health department's definition of a major injury.

Percent of residents who lose too much weight (long stay)

This quality measure is the percentage of long-stay residents who have a weight loss of 5% in the last month or 10% in the last six months, when they weren't on a physician-prescribed weight-loss program.

Data source:

- **K0300** (weight loss)

K0300: Weight Loss

K0300. Weight Loss	
Enter Code	**Loss of 5% or more in the last month or loss of 10% or more in last 6 months** 0. **No** or unknown 1. **Yes, on** physician-prescribed weight-loss regimen 2. **Yes, not on** physician-prescribed weight-loss regimen

If K0300 = 2, then the resident is counted as having a weight loss of 5% or more in the last month or 10% or more in the last 6 months.

Tricky parts

Weight loss calculations have to be done with actual values, including decimals. This is different than what is reported on the MDS, which only uses whole numbers.

Unmeasurable residents: If a resident can't be weight because of extreme pain, immobility, risk of pathological fractures, and so on, then you should code a dash (-) and document the rationale in the medical record. This resident will then be excluded from the quality measure calculations.

K0710 (percent intake by artificial route)

Lookback period: 7 days

K0710: Percent Intake by Artificial Route

Complete K0710 only if Column 1 and/or Column 2 are checked for K0510A and/or K0510B.

K0710. Percent Intake by Artificial Route - Complete K0710 only if Column 1 and/or Column 2 are checked for K0510A and/or K0510B	2. While a Resident	3. During Entire 7 Days
2. While a Resident Performed *while a resident* of this facility and within the *last 7 days* **3. During Entire 7 Days** Performed during the entire *last 7 days*	↓ Enter Codes ↓	
A. Proportion of total calories the resident received through parenteral or tube feeding 1. 25% or less 2. 26-50% 3. 51% or more	☐	☐
B. Average fluid intake per day by IV or tube feeding 1. 500 cc/day or less 2. 501 cc/day or more	☐	☐

This quality measure is the percentage of total calories that a resident received through parenteral or tube feeding. This item also captures the total number of calories through parenteral or tube feeding and the average fluid intake per day by IV or tube feeding. You can code for whether the parenteral or tube feeding was performed while the patient was a resident of the nursing facility and whether it happened during the entire 7-day lookback period.

K0710-A: proportion of total calories through parenteral or tube feeding

K0710-B: average fluid intake per day by IV or tube feeding

70

Tricky parts

When calculating the feeding tube and IV intake over the 7-day lookback period, you should add up all the feedings and divide by 7, even if the resident didn't have any artificial intake on some days.

Special Care High or a Special Care Low: Under the Patient Driven Payment Model (PDPM), a resident can be sorted into the Special Care High or a Special Care Low case-mix group if they received either:

- **K0710-A = 3**: 51% or more of total calories through tube feeding
- **K0710-A = 2 and K0710B = 2**: 26%–50% of total calories through tube feeding and 501cc per day or more of fluid intake via tube

for the entirety of the 7-day lookback period.

Section M (skin conditions)

	M0300. Current Number of Unhealed Pressure Ulcers/Injuries at Each Stage
	A. Stage 1: Intact skin with non-blanchable redness of a localized area usually over a bony prominence. Darkly pigmented skin may not have a visible blanching; in dark skin tones only it may appear with persistent blue or purple hues
Enter Number ☐	**1. Number of Stage 1 pressure injuries**
	B. Stage 2: Partial thickness loss of dermis presenting as a shallow open ulcer with a red or pink wound bed, without slough. May also present as an intact or open/ruptured blister
Enter Number ☐	**1. Number of Stage 2 pressure ulcers -** If 0 → Skip to M0300C, Stage 3
Enter Number ☐	**2. Number of these Stage 2 pressure ulcers that were present upon admission/entry or reentry -** enter how many were noted at the time of admission/entry or reentry
	C. Stage 3: Full thickness tissue loss. Subcutaneous fat may be visible but bone, tendon or muscle is not exposed. Slough may be present but does not obscure the depth of tissue loss. May include undermining and tunneling
Enter Number ☐	**1. Number of Stage 3 pressure ulcers -** If 0 → Skip to M0300D, Stage 4
Enter Number ☐	**2. Number of these Stage 3 pressure ulcers that were present upon admission/entry or reentry** - enter how many were noted at the time of admission/entry or reentry
	D. Stage 4: Full thickness tissue loss with exposed bone, tendon or muscle. Slough or eschar may be present on some parts of the wound bed. Often includes undermining and tunneling
Enter Number ☐	**1. Number of Stage 4 pressure ulcers -** If 0 → Skip to M0300E, Unstageable - Non-removable dressing/device
Enter Number ☐	**2. Number of these Stage 4 pressure ulcers that were present upon admission/entry or reentry -** enter how many were noted at the time of admission/entry or reentry
	E. Unstageable - Non-removable dressing/device: Known but not stageable due to non-removable dressing/device
Enter Number ☐	**1. Number of unstageable pressure ulcers/injuries due to non-removable dressing/device -** If 0 → Skip to M0300F, Unstageable - Slough and/or eschar
Enter Number ☐	**2. Number of these unstageable pressure ulcers/injuries that were present upon admission/entry or reentry -** enter how many were noted at the time of admission/entry or reentry
	F. Unstageable - Slough and/or eschar: Known but not stageable due to coverage of wound bed by slough and/or eschar
Enter Number ☐	**1. Number of unstageable pressure ulcers due to coverage of wound bed by slough and/or eschar -** If 0 → Skip to M0300G, Unstageable - Deep tissue injury
Enter Number ☐	**2. Number of these unstageable pressure ulcers that were present upon admission/entry or reentry -** enter how many were noted at the time of admission/entry or reentry
	G. Unstageable - Deep tissue injury:
Enter Number ☐	**1. Number of unstageable pressure injuries presenting as deep tissue injury -** If 0 → Skip to M1030, Number of Venous and Arterial Ulcers
Enter Number ☐	**2. Number of these unstageable pressure injuries that were present upon admission/entry or reentry -** enter how many were noted at the time of admission/entry or reentry

Percent of high-risk residents with pressure ulcers (long stay)

Reporting period: 3 months

This quality measure is the percentage of long-stay, high-risk residents who at least one stage 2, 3, 4, or unstageable pressure injury.

A high-risk resident must have at least one of these three criteria:

- **G0110-A1** = 3, 4, 7, or 8: impaired bed mobility, self-performance
- **G0110-B1** = 3, 4, 7, or 8: impaired transfer, self-performance
- **B0100** = 1: comatose
- **I5600** = 1: malnutrition or at risk of malnutrition

Tricky parts

This quality measure doesn't include stage 1 pressure injuries. It also doesn't include pressure injuries from the admission assessment or the 5-day assessment, since whatever pressure injuries the resident had at that time occurred before the nursing home got the resident.

Percent of residents with pressure ulcers that are new or worsened (short stay)

Reporting period: 12 months

This quality measure is the percentage of Medicare part A, type 1 SNF stay residents who have stage 2, 3, or 4 pressure ulcers that are new or worsened since admission.

How to identify Medicare Part A (type 1 only) SNF stays

A resident's **5-day PPS assessment** and **discharge assessment** defines whether or not they had a Medicare Part A (type 1 only) SNF stay. The assessments can also be:

- a standalone Part A PPS discharge
- a Part A PPS discharge combined with an OBRA discharge assessment.

If a resident has multiple Medicare Part (type 1 only) stays during the 12-month reporting period, then all the eligible stays are included in the quality measure.

Covariates

The covariates for this quality measure are:

- Limited bed mobility, self-performance
- Bowel incontinence
- Diabetes
- Peripheral vascular disease or peripheral arterial disease
- Low body mass index

Tricky parts

This quality measure only takes into consideration stage 2, 3, and 4 pressure injuries. It doesn't include unstageable ulcers. Here are some other common scenarios that can be difficult to code correctly.

Changes in pressure injury stage

Increase in numerical stage: If the resident had a pressure injury during admission or re-entry, but then the pressure injury increased in stage during the resident's stay, then you should code the pressure injury as the higher stage and the higher stage as "not present on admission."

Injury becomes unstageable: If the resident had a pressure injury during admission or re-entry, but then the pressure injury becomes unstageable (M0300F), then you should code the injury as M0300F and "not present on admission."

Unstageable to numerical: If the resident had an unstageable pressure injury on admission or re-entry, but then becomes stageable later, then you should code the first numerical stage as the time as "not present on admission." If this numerical stage later increases, then the higher stage is also coded as "not present on admission."

Hospitalized residents

Resident with a pressure injury that he acquired in the nursing home: If a resident already has a pressure injury that was **acquired in the facility**, but then goes to the hospital, returns, and comes back with the same pressure in injury, then you should code it as "not present on admission" upon re-entry. This is because the pressure injury was present before his hospitalization.

Resident with a pressure injury that he had before he was admitted to the nursing home: If a resident already has a pressure injury that was **present on admission**, then goes to the hospital, returns, and comes back with the same pressure injury, then you should code it as "present on admission" because it was originally acquired outside the nursing facility and it hasn't changed.

Pressure injury that increases in numerical stage or becomes unstageable: If a resident who already has a pressure injury goes to the hospital, comes back, and

the pressure injury increases in numerical stage or becomes unstageable, then it should be coded as "present on admission" upon re-entry.

Pressure injury that becomes unstageable, but later becomes stageable and the numerical stage is higher than before: If a resident who already has a pressure injury goes to the hospital, comes back, and the pressure injury becomes unstageable, but later recovers a bit and the unstageable injury becomes stageable, then you should code it as "not present on admission" if the numerical stage had increased.

Merging pressure injuries

Two pressure injuries merge: If a resident has two pressure injuries that were present on admission, and the two injuries merge, then code the merged pressure injury as "present on admission."

Two pressure injuries merge and increase in numerical stage or become unstageable: If a resident has two pressure injuries that were present on admission, and the two injuries merge, and the merged injury increases in numerical stage or becomes unstageable, then code the merged pressure injury as "not present on admission."

Section N (medications)

Percent of residents who newly received an antipsychotic medication (short stay)

This quality measure is the percentage of short-stay residents who newly received an antipsychotic medication. This means that they are on an anti-psychotic medication during the target assessment, but they weren't during the initial assessment.

Data sources:

- **N0410-A** (anti-psychotic medication)

N0410. Medications Received	
Indicate the number of DAYS the resident received the following medications by pharmacological classification, not how it is used, during the last 7 days or since admission/entry or reentry if less than 7 days. Enter "0" if medication was not received by the resident during the last 7 days	
Enter Days ☐	A. Antipsychotic
Enter Days ☐	B. Antianxiety
Enter Days ☐	C. Antidepressant
Enter Days ☐	D. Hypnotic
Enter Days ☐	E. Anticoagulant (e.g., warfarin, heparin, or low-molecular weight heparin)
Enter Days ☐	F. Antibiotic
Enter Days ☐	G. Diuretic
Enter Days ☐	H. Opioid

Calculations

If N0410-A (anti-psychotic medication) = 1–7, then the resident is counted as having received an anti-psychotic medication. Residents with the following conditions are excluded from this quality measure:

- **I5250** (Huntington's disease)
- **I5350** (Tourette's syndrome)
- **I6000** (schizophrenia)

Tricky parts

A diagnosis of dementia does **not** exclude a resident from being in this quality measure.

Prevalence of antianxiety/hypnotic use (long stay)

This quality measure is the prevalence of long-stay residents who use anti-anxiety or hypnotic drugs but who don't have psychosis or a related condition.

> Note: This is **not** the same as the "residents who used an anti-anxiety or hypnotic medication" quality measure. That is a quality measure used for public reporting. It also doesn't have a covariant applied to it.

Data source:

- **N0410-B** (anti-anxiety medication)
- **N0410-D** (hypnotic medication)

Calculations

This is the list of diagnoses that exclude a resident from this quality measure:

- **E0100-A** (hallucinations)
- **E0100-B** (delusions)
- **I5250** (Huntington's disease)
- **I5350** (Tourette's syndrome)
- **I5700** (anxiety disorder)
- **I5950** (psychotic disorder)
- **I6000** (schizophrenia)
- **I5900** (manic depression, bipolar disease)
- **I6100** (post-traumatic stress disorder)

Tricky parts

Residents with dementia may chronically experience delusions or hallucinations. Nursing home staff often overlook delusions (E0100B) in these residents because they've become desensitized to their behaviors. It's still important to code these behaviors into the resident's medical record.

Percent of long-stay residents who received an antipsychotic medication

This quality measure is the percentage of long-stay residents who received an anti-psychotic medication and who didn't have psychosis or a related condition.

Data source:

- **N0410-A** (anti-psychotic medication)

If N0410-A (anti-psychotic medication) = 1–7, then the resident is counted as having received an anti-psychotic medication. Residents with the following conditions are excluded from this quality measure:

- **I5250** (Huntington's disease)
- **I5350** (Tourette's syndrome)
- **I6000** (schizophrenia)

Tricky parts

The exclusion criteria does not include diagnoses in item I8000. For example, if a resident has Huntington's disease and the coder puts it in I8000 instead of I5250, then the resident will erroneously be put in this quality measure.

Section P (restraints and alarms)

Percent of residents who were physically restrained (long stay)

This quality measure is the percentage of long-stay residents who are physically restrained on a daily basis.

Data source:

- **P0100-B** (trunk restraint used in bed)
- **P0100-C** (limb restraint used in bed)
- **P0100-E** (trunk restraint used in chair or out of bed)
- **P0100-F** (limb restraint used in chair or out of bed)
- **P0100-G** (chair prevents rising used in chair or out of bed)

Section P	Restraints and Alarms

P0100. Physical Restraints

Physical restraints are any manual method or physical or mechanical device, material or equipment attached or adjacent to the resident's body that the individual cannot remove easily which restricts freedom of movement or normal access to one's body

Coding:	↓ Enter Codes in Boxes
	Used in Bed
	☐ A. Bed rail
	☐ B. Trunk restraint
	☐ C. Limb restraint
0. Not used	☐ D. Other
1. Used less than daily	**Used in Chair or Out of Bed**
2. Used daily	☐ E. Trunk restraint
	☐ F. Limb restraint
	☐ G. Chair prevents rising
	☐ H. Other

Tricky parts

This quality measure is only triggered if the P0100-B, C, E, F, or G are coded as 2 (used daily). P0100-A (bed rail) is not included in this quality measure.

Geri chairs: Residents who have no voluntary or involuntary movements can be put in Geri chairs. It is not considered a physical restraint.

Lap boards: A chair with an unlocked lap board could be coded as "chair prevents rising" if the resident can't easily remove the lap board.

Side rails: If a resident has no movement, then side rails are not considered restraints. Although, they probably shouldn't have side rails in the first place.

Wheeled walkers: Enclosed-frame wheeled walkers may be considered restraints if the resident can't get out of the walker by removing the tray or opening the gate.

Locked unit or secure unit: A locked or secure unit is not a restraint. It is a building that the resident has the freedom to move around in.

Chapter 13: QAPI and QAA programs

A nursing home's quality assurance and performance improvement (QAPI) or quality assessment and assurance (QAA) program must monitor their facility's clinical care and identify problems with its performance. Here are some tips on running a successful QAPI program.

Public quality measures and consumer interest

Some quality measures are publicly reported on the Compare website, formerly Nursing Home Compare. Residents, family members, visitors, and potential clients all look at those numbers. The staff members, especially the medical director, physician, and administrator, should be kept up to date on quality measures, the facility's scores, areas that need improvement, efforts to improve the low-scoring areas, and how to talk about them. For example, the raw statistic might be that "12 percent of high-risk residents have pressure injuries." When a family member asks about that, you can say that "88% of our residents are free from pressure injury."

Train staff in MDS data accuracy

Inaccuracies in MDS coding can distort your nursing home's quality scores, as well as lead to inaccurate care plans and poor clinical outcomes. Rules for MDS change a lot, so it's important that staff go to refresher training periodically.

Long-Term Care Facility Resident Assessment Instrument User's Manual

CMS will regularly update their Long-Term Care Facility Resident Assessment Instrument User's Manual. It might be useful to put a copy of it on the nursing desk or break room, as well as regularly re-reprinting that copy.

Quality measures expert

A nursing home should designate one person as the quality measures expert. This person should be trained in MDS, the SNF Quality Reporting Program (QRP), and quality measures in general. This person can be responsible for monitoring the quality measure scores and training the rest of the staff in quality measures.